A SPA OF YOUR OWN

recipes for refreshing skin, hair, and body treatments

Stephanie Tourles

The mission of Storey Publishing is to serve our customers
by publishing practical information that encourages personal independence
in harmony with the environment.

Edited by Deborah Balmuth and Robin Catalano
Cover design by Wendy Palitz
Cover background illustrations by Alexandra Eckhardt
Cover image art © Juliette Borda
Text design and production by Susan Bernier

Printed in the United States by Lake Book
10 9 8 7 6 5 4 3 2 1

ISBN 1-58017-888-X

Introduction:
Let Go of the Guilt

The word *pamper* is a verb meaning "to gratify the wishes of, especially by catering to physical comforts." It also means "to spoil, coddle, humor, indulge, or caress." Sounds like pampering is something most of us could use more of in these stressful times.

We're all so very busy, busy, busy. Buzzing around like worker bees, tending to everyone else's needs and ignoring our own. Do you work all day caring for children or elderly parents, or work outside the home in a 40- to 60-hour-per-week career? Are you a full-time student? Isn't it ecstasy to know that after you finish all that work, you get to grocery shop, cook dinner, do laundry, clean the house, pay the bills, mow the lawn, fix the car, and meet with the insurance agent? Sure it is! Who needs personal time?

As if life wasn't busy enough before technology exploded onto the scene, now we're expected to be super-people. Living life at breakneck speed can make us feel as if we're on a wild roller-coaster ride that won't stop. We can't continue to work faster and faster and process more and more information and still function as normal, happy, healthy human beings. Needless to say, most of us are frazzled. We need a break . . . to catch our breath, to regain our health, to restore our natural rhythms, to enjoy the meaningful moments in life that have gone by the wayside because we're so busy. In a word, we need *pampering.*

It's not a dirty word that should make you feel guilty. You deserve a bit of pampering. I'm sure you've earned it.

By pampering yourself, you don't have to take an entire day off and loaf around (though that's advisable from time to time); you can simply integrate small moments of pampering into your everyday life. This book is filled with simple ways to de-stress and unwind, to find more pleasure and joy, and to look and feel better. These invaluable tips will help you enjoy more "you" time. When you're happier and calmer, radiant from the inside out, glowing with health and beauty, believe me, those around you will sit up and take notice.

So go ahead, pamper yourself . . . you're worth it!

**Blessings of health and happiness
to you and yours,**
Stephanie L. Tourles

Information and Cautions

Most of the ingredients mentioned in this book, including essential oils and herbs, can be found in natural-food or health-food stores. Natural product and herbal mail-order suppliers are also a good place to look.

When using any new ingredient for the first time, it's always best to try a patch test. Apply a bit of the ingredient or formula to the inside of your arm, and allow it to remain for 24 hours. If any signs of allergic response — redness, itching, or other skin irritation — occur, discontinue use immediately. In addition, be sure to use caution in handling pure essential oils. Because they are highly concentrated, they can cause adverse skin reactions. Always use a dropper when measuring essential oils, and do not use more than recommended; more can be dangerous, not better. Keep all ingredients out of the reach of children and pets.

Get Steamed

An herbal facial steam will hydrate your skin and allow your pores to perspire and breathe. As the steam penetrates your skin, the various herbs will soften its surface, act as an astringent, and aid in healing skin lesions. Also, any clogging from dirt or makeup will be loosened for easy removal afterward.

Herbal steams can be used regularly by those with normal, dry, or oily skin. Those of you with sensitive skin, dilated capillaries, rosacea, or sunburned skin, however, should abstain. Always cleanse your skin before steaming.

Steams for Pore Perfection

To prepare a facial steam, boil 4 cups of distilled water (and vinegar, if the recipe calls for it). Remove from the heat, add herbs, cover, and allow to steep for about 5 minutes. Place the pot in a safe, stable place where you can sit comfortably for about 10 minutes. Use a bath towel to create a tent over your head, your shoulders, and the steaming herb pot; allow 10 to 12 inches between the steaming herb pot and your face to avoid burning your skin. Close your eyes, breathe deeply, and relax.

All the herbs in the following blends are in dried form. If you're using fresh herbs, double the quantity.

- **For Normal or Oily Skin:** 1 teaspoon yarrow, 1 teaspoon sage, 1 teaspoon rosemary, and 1 teaspoon peppermint.

- **For Normal or Dry Skin:** 1 teaspoon orange flowers, 2 teaspoons comfrey leaves, and 1 teaspoon elder flowers.

- **For All Skin Types:** 1 teaspoon calendula, 1 teaspoon chamomile, 1 teaspoon raspberry leaves, 1 teaspoon peppermint, and 1 teaspoon strawberry leaves.

- **Wrinkle Chaser:** 1 tablespoon crushed fennel seeds and 2 drops essential oil of rose or rose geranium. Add the essential oil to the water immediately before you steam your face.

Aromatherapy to Relax or Recharge

The word *aroma,* meaning "a pleasant or agreeable odor arising from spices, plants, or flowers," combined with the word *therapy,* or "the remedial treatment of a disease or other physical or mental disorder," gives us the true definition of the word *aromatherapy:* a healing modality that involves the use of aromatic essences or essential oils of plants.

Incorporating essential oils into your life is a pleasurable way to enhance your physical, emotional, and spiritual well-being. Aromatherapy can beautify your complexion, reduce stress, stimulate creativity, lull you to sleep, and pep you up, as well as help heal severe burns and reduce scar formation.

Strike a Balance

• **One of the easiest** and most pleasant ways to benefit from aromatherapy is in the bath. At day's end, add 3 to 6 drops of your favorite gentle essential oil, such as lavender,

Roman or German chamomile, or clary sage, to a full tub of water and swish with your hands to blend. Slip into the water and breathe deeply. Relax . . .

• **Intensify the potency of your peppermint tea.** Give it a little zing by adding 1 or 2 drops of essential oil of peppermint. Inhale the invigorating steam. This tea is super for a midmorning pick-me-up, and it's wonderful at relieving a stuffy head or case of indigestion. Makes your breath minty-fresh, too!

• **To ease the pain of muscle cramps,** sore tendons, arthritis, or overexertion in general, the clean, fresh, lemony scent of essential oil of *Eucalyptus citriodora* makes a soothing addition to massage oil. Add 10 to 15 drops of essential oil to ½ cup of almond, hazelnut, grapeseed, or soybean oil; mix well; and massage away the discomfort. Enlist the help of a partner or good friend if possible, and promise to return the favor.

Harmony Aroma Oil

Choose a blend to suit your particular emotional and physical needs. *Caution:* These formulas are for inhalation only. Do not apply directly to the skin; they may cause irritation.

Calming Blend: For stress, restlessness, or insomnia, or cold, dry weather, use ½ teaspoon lavender, ½ teaspoon neroli, ½ teaspoon clary sage, and ½ teaspoon bergamot essential oils.

Cooling Blend: For irritability, impatience, fiery disposition, or chaos, or if the weather outside is hot and uncomfortable and your skin is extra sensitive and itchy, use ½ teaspoon lavender, ½ teaspoon jasmine, ½ teaspoon Roman chamomile, and ½ teaspoon spearmint essential oils.

Stimulating Blend: If you're feeling slow and lethargic, in need of an energetic lift, and maybe a bit congested, or if the weather is dreary, cool, and damp, use ½ teaspoon cinnamon, ½ teaspoon orange, ½ teaspoon ginger, and ½ teaspoon cypress essential oils.

Combine the blend of your choice with 1 tablespoon pure, unrefined almond, jojoba, or hazelnut oil in a 2-ounce, dark glass bottle and cap tightly. Shake your formula vigorously twice daily for seven days. To use, place a few drops on a handkerchief or tissue and inhale as needed, or inhale directly from the bottle.

Make a Splash

Nothing is more refreshing to hot summer skin than a chilled splash of a freshly made natural skin toner. Like a summer breeze that soothes your parched skin and senses, these lightly scented toners can be customized to your skin type and fragrance preference.

Give Your Skin a "Drink"

Natural skin toners have been used for centuries to refresh, pamper, and gently scent the skin and air. The following toner recipes can be applied as a splash, as a light mist from a spray bottle, or with cotton balls. Use at any time or right after cleansing to remove traces of cleanser and prepare your skin for moisturizer. Store in the refrigerator and discard after one week unless otherwise indicated.

• **For normal or oily skin,** brew a cup of strong peppermint or lemon balm tea. Chill it, and use it to remove excess oil and shine from your skin.

• **For itchy, rashy skin,** pour a cup of boiling water over 1 teaspoon of crushed fennel seeds. Steep for 10 minutes. Strain and chill.

• **For all skin types,** brew a cup of strong chamomile tea, chill, and use to soften and moisturize. This is particularly good to use during the winter, when skin dehydrates and chaps easily.

• **For normal and dry skin,** add 1 tablespoon of vegetable glycerin to ½ cup of rose water. The glycerin will act as a humectant and draw water vapor from the air to your skin. This makes a super, light floral summer moisturizer that can be stored in the refrigerator for up to six months. Shake before each use.

Polish Your Body

A cosmetic scrub is used to remove dry, dead cells from the surface of the skin. It can be used on all skin types except those with acne, thread (spider) veins, or extreme sensitivity; it may be too irritating for these. The recipes below will leave your skin softer, sleeker, and more refined, in prime condition to absorb an application of moisturizer.

Natural Scrubs and Salt Rubs

• **For dry or sensitive skin:** In a small bowl, combine 1 tablespoon of instant, powdered whole milk, 1 scant tablespoon of ground oatmeal, and enough water to form a spreadable paste. Allow to thicken for 1 minute. Massage onto your face and throat, avoiding the eye area. Rinse. This formula may be used daily in place of soap to gently cleanse your face and body. It will not irritate or dry your skin.

• **Especially for men** or those with thick, oily skin: In a small bowl, combine 1 teaspoon of ground oatmeal, 1 teaspoon of finely ground almond meal, 1 teaspoon of fine sea salt, and ½ teaspoon of powdered peppermint or rosemary leaves with enough of your favorite herbal astringent to form a spreadable paste. Allow to thicken for 1 minute. Massage gently onto your face and throat, avoiding the eye area. Rinse. This blend is particularly good to use on the chest, back, or shoulders if minor pimple breakouts tend to occur.

• **For all skin types:** In a small bowl, combine ¼ cup of sea salt (or plain sugar) with ¼ cup of warmed coconut or olive oil. Stir together. Gently massage onto your body with your hands or a mitt using light but firm pressure. Continue massaging until a rosy glow appears. Rinse with warm water, then towel-dry. This blend is beneficial for those suffering from severely dry skin: It will effectively remove the top layer of dead skin cells, allowing for proper moisturizer absorption. *Note:* This scrub should not be used on your face or immediately after shaving any area of your body; it could cause stinging and irritation.

• **For all skin types, especially dehydrated:** In a small bowl, combine 1 tablespoon of finely ground sunflower seed meal with 1 tablespoon of applesauce. Gently massage this paste onto your face and throat. Let it remain for 10 minutes so that the oils of the sunflower seeds can be released and absorbed into your thirsty skin. Rinse with warm water, and then pat dry.

 Grinding Ingredients

To grind oatmeal, sunflower seeds, almonds, dried herbs, and similar ingredients, I like to use a regular coffee grinder specifically reserved for cosmetic making. A blender or food processor works well for batches larger than 1 cup. Either method will create a fine, powderlike consistency.

Step Lively

"My feet are killing me!" Do you ever say that at the end of a long day? Whether you're a construction worker, an athlete, a stay-at-home parent, or a fashion model, your feet take a lot of abuse. Most people stuff their feet into ill-fitting shoes and suffer from cramped and strained arches, heel pain, hammertoes, bunions, calluses, corns, and toe cramps.

If you want your feet to provide you with years of uninterrupted service, treat them with the utmost care. Daily hygiene and a few foot exercises go a long way. Do keep in mind though, that 10 to 15 minutes of foot exercise every day will not do any good if you continue to wear ill-fitting shoes that constrict movement and force your feet into unnatural shapes.

Exercise Those "Dogs"

The following foot, ankle, and toe exercises can be performed anytime you feel the need to stretch and release tension. If you can't slip off your shoes discreetly during the day, then perform the exercises when you get home from work or finish your daily errands. Slip your body into something more comfortable and slip your feet out of something uncomfortable (your shoes). Relax and unwind. A nice cup of soothing herbal tea, sipped while you do your exercises, tastes especially good, hot or cold!

• **Footsie Roller Massage:** Wooden footsie rollers have been around for many years. They come in all shapes and sizes, from single to double or triple rollers. Some are hand-held, and others sit on the floor. I particularly like the kind with raised ridges going from one end to the other; these are both stimulating and relaxing to my feet. If you don't have a footsie roller, a wooden rolling pin can be used. Simply place the footsie roller or rolling pin on the floor and, while bearing down comfortably, roll the entire length of your foot over the tool, back and forth. Repeat, concentrating on your arches. Do this for 5 to 10 minutes per foot. This exercise relieves fatigue and cramping, especially in your arches.

• **The Golf Ball Roll:** This exercise is recommended by Carol Frey, M.D., director of the Orthopedic Foot and Ankle Center in Manhattan Beach, California. "Roll a golf ball under the ball of your foot for 2 minutes. A great massage for the bottom of the foot, recommended for people with plantar fasciitis (heel pain), arch strain, or foot cramps."

• **Point and Flex:** This will stretch and strengthen everything from your knees down. Sit on the floor, legs out in front of you and palms facing down at your sides. Point your toes as hard as you can and hold for 5 seconds; then flex your foot up as hard as you can and hold for 5 seconds. Repeat 10 times. If cramps occur, cut back on your repetitions and gradually work up to 10.

• **Rubber-Band Big Toe Stretches:** These are helpful for bunions or toe cramps resulting from improperly fitting shoes. Sit on the floor with your legs stretched out in front of you and your palms on the floor beside or behind you, or sit in a chair with your feet flat on the floor. Place a thick, moderately stiff rubber band around your big toes and pull your feet away from each other. Hold for 5 to 10 seconds, and then relax. Repeat 10 to 20 times. If this hurts, or if you have arthritis or bunions in advanced stages, do only as many as you can. Gradually increase as your toes gain strength.

Nourish Your Hair

Healthy, shiny, bouncy hair is a reflection of proper nourishment and a healthy lifestyle. Even if you use the highest-quality natural shampoos, conditioners, and styling aids, the condition of your hair will still suffer if your diet is lacking in necessary nutrients. If your hair seems lackluster, try modifying your diet.

How to Have Healthy Hair

• **Eat more protein** if your locks are limp, lifeless, and slow growing. Good sources of protein include eggs, lean meats and fish, beans and seeds, whole grains, and low-fat dairy or soy products.

• **Get your ABCs.** Vitamins are vital to the health of your hair and scalp. Good sources of vitamin A include cod liver oil; red, yellow, and orange vegetables and fruits; spirulina; egg yolks; and deep green leafy vegetables. Good sources of vitamin C include citrus fruits, deep green leafy vegetables, rose hips, tomatoes, berries, pineapple, apples, persimmons, cherries, bell and hot peppers, papayas, and currants. Good sources of vitamin B include lean beef, poultry, egg yolks, liver, milk, brewer's yeast, whole grains, alfalfa, nuts and seeds, soy products, deep green leafy vegetables, spirulina, wheat germ, molasses, peas, and beans.

• **Cut back on caffeine,** alcohol, refined sugar and flour, and junky snacks. These empty-calorie foods deplete your body's stores of vitamins B and C.

• **Include iodine, sulfur, zinc, and silica in your diet.** These four minerals are essential for proper hair health. Good sources of iodine include all types of fish, spirulina, sunflower seeds, iodized salt, and sea salt. Good sources of sulfur include turnips, dandelion greens, radishes, horse-radish, string beans, onions, garlic, cabbage, celery, kale, watercress, fish, lean meats, eggs, and asparagus. Good sources of zinc include spirulina, barley grass, alfalfa, kelp, wheat germ, pumpkin seeds, whole grains, brewer's yeast, milk, eggs, oysters, nuts, and beans. Good sources of silica include horsetail, spirulina, nettles, dandelion root, alfalfa, kelp, flaxseeds, oat straw, barley grass, wheat grass, apples, berries, burdock roots, beets, onions, almonds, sunflower seeds, and grapes.

Rapunzel's Favorite Herb Tea

I won't guarantee that this tea will make you sprout hair as long and lush as Rapunzel's, but this mineral-rich brew is a delightful way to nourish your hair from the inside out. This recipe uses dried herbs and will yield 2 cups of tea.

½ teaspoon horsetail
½ teaspoon raspberry leaves
½ teaspoon nettles
½ teaspoon oat straw

1 teaspoon peppermint
2 cups boiling water
Honey or lemon to taste (optional)

Add the herbs to the boiling water, then remove from heat. Cover and steep for 5 to 10 minutes. Strain. Add honey or lemon to taste, if desired. Sip slowly and enjoy!

Top 10 Healing Foods

If you really want to pamper your mind and body, then partaking of these top 10 nutritionally dynamic foods is just what the doctor ordered. They'll help balance your moods; restore your energy; increase your stamina; nourish your hair, skin, and nails; and boost your immune system. They're delicious to boot!

Eat for Vibrant Health

• **Beans,** beans, the magical food — the more you eat them, the better your mood! It's true: Beans are high in the B vitamins, known mood stabilizers. They're also high in complex carbohydrates, magnesium, iron, zinc, and fiber. A cup or so a day is recommended.

• **Broccoli** is a nutritional powerhouse. Just ½ cup several times per week delivers most of your daily required vitamin C, a dollop of vitamin A and the B complex, and plenty of minerals, especially calcium; it's also rich in fiber.

• **Oranges** are chock-full of skin-healthy, cold-fighting vitamin C, soluble and insoluble fiber, bioflavonoids, folate, and potassium. Consume one or more per day.

• **Apples** are tasty, easy to carry, and thirst quenching. They're rich in soluble and insoluble fiber, potassium, and trace minerals. An apple a day sure won't hurt!

• **Bananas** are high in natural sugar and are self-contained packages of quick, healthy energy. They contain a fair amount of B-complex vitamins, vitamin C, and soluble and insoluble fibers and are a good source of potassium and magnesium. Consume a few of these energy-boosting fruits each week.

• **Water** can temporarily give you a feeling of fullness, hydrate your skin, keep your organs operating smoothly, and flush toxins out of your body. Drink 8 to 12 eight-ounce glasses each day, depending upon your level of activity.

• **Sesame seeds** are little storehouses of highly absorbable calcium and magnesium. They're also high in fiber and trace minerals. Look in health food stores for raw, unhulled seeds or jars of sesame tahini (sesame paste). Two tablespoons per day of seeds or paste will make a major contribution toward your daily mineral requirement.

- **Shellfish** deliver a powerful nutritional punch. Shrimp, scallops, clams, crab, abalone, lobster, snails, crayfish, oysters, conch, and prawns are high in beauty nutrients such as protein, B-complex vitamins, iron, iodine, zinc, and copper. Two servings per week are recommended.

- **Garlic,** a potent antioxidant, can cut cholesterol, ward off infection, soothe a sore throat, protect your heart, and kill athlete's foot fungus. An ounce of fresh garlic contains a good helping of vitamin C, thiamin (vitamin B_1), potassium, sulfur, and iron. Eat a clove or two every day.

- **Salmon** is the king of flavor and a rich source of beneficial omega-3 fats, which have been determined to help prevent heart problems and lessen the symptoms of arthritis and PMS. Eating one or more servings of salmon per week is recommended.

Five (Almost) Free Daily Rituals for Beautiful Skin

Skin care shouldn't be a complex chore. It should be simple, natural, and basic. And if a few of these straightforward skin-care rituals are free for the asking, then so much the better!

Tried-and-True Treatments

• **Cleansing Routine:** A beauty must! Cleanse your skin twice daily (only once if your skin is dry) using a mild, natural, inexpensive cleanser designed for your skin type. Add a couple of drops of essential oil of rose, spearmint, or orange to your cleanser to boost its cleansing effect and aromatic quality. Cleansing your skin before going to bed is especially important, because your body excretes toxins through your skin as you sleep. If facial pores are clogged with makeup and dirt, breakouts can occur. If you perspire a lot in your line of work or exercise heavily, then rinse off and massage your body with a coarse cloth or loofah before retiring to remove salt and dead-skin buildup. Your skin needs to breathe while you sleep!

• **Exercise:** Try to exercise outside, to help oxygenate your cells with fresh air and facilitate waste removal through your skin. Exercises such as walking, biking, in-line skating, and weight lifting improve cardiovascular fitness and muscular endurance, which translates into increased energy and a rosy complexion. If you live in a city, try to find a green space — a park or a greenway — in which to exercise. If city streets, with their attendant pollution, are your only outdoor option, exercising in a gym may be a better alternative.

• **Sleep, Blissful Sleep:** I don't care what else you do to your skin, if you are sleep deprived your skin will look sallow, dull, tired, and saggy; with your puffy eyes, you will resemble a frog prince or princess. And of course, your energy level will be less than desirable. Sleep: It's the best-kept skin-care secret there is!

• **Sunlight:** Ten to 15 minutes unprotected exposure to sunlight several times a week is essential to the health of your bones and skin. It helps your body absorb calcium, because the skin can convert the sun's rays into vitamin D. Sun exposure helps heal eczema, psoriasis, and acne, and it energizes your body. Plus those warm rays just make you feel good all over. If your dermatologist advises you to avoid the sun entirely, other sources of vitamin D include egg yolks, fish liver oil, vitamin-D-supplemented soy or cow's milk, organ meats, salmon, sardines, and herring.

• **Water:** What goes in must go out, and water helps move everything along. Impurities not disposed of in a timely manner via the internal organs of elimination (such as the kidneys, liver, lungs, and large intestine) will find an alternate exit, namely your skin, sometimes referred to as the "third kidney." Pimples and rashes may develop as your body tries to unload its wastes through your skin. Eight to 12 eight-ounce glasses of pure water a day combined with a fibrous diet will help cleanse your body of toxins and keep your colon functioning as it should. Water also keeps your skin hydrated and moisturized, so drink up!

De-stress and Relax

Seems like everyone is so very busy these days, no matter what their job description. I've spoken with many stay-at-home parents, career men and women, elderly folks, and students, asking them for their favorite methods to relax and de-stress after a hectic day. Try some of these ways to unwind.

• **"If I am stressed,"** I like to go for a long walk, because it helps me unwind."

• **"If stressed while at work,"** I try to breathe in deeply and then exhale slowly."

• **"I find taking a leisurely bath"** with oils or a bubble bath to be very soothing."

• **"I have a monthly facial."**

• **"To relax,** I do stretching exercises for about 15 minutes with my eyes closed while listening to calming music."

• **"My greatest de-stressor** is usually a creative pursuit. I make quilts and garden, primarily. The final products are lasting delights that I cherish."

• **"Cooking relaxes my mind and body.** Eating what I've prepared is great, too!"

• **"Sipping a glass of wine** while reading a good book chases the day's cares away."

• **"Good heart-to-heart conversation,** a romantic candlelight dinner, and a walk on the beach at sunset with my husband is my idea of heaven."

• **"I like to putter in my garden,** feel the soil, and pull weeds after work."

Soothe Your Soles

If your nerves are frayed, your energy is running on empty, and your feet have seen better days, by all means partake of an aromatherapy foot massage. It will soothe your spirits, reduce stress, put spring in your step, and soften your feet. What's good for the body is good for the "sole"!

Techniques of Foot Massage

Here are some standard foot-massage techniques that a professional nail technician might perform on a client during a pedicure. If you do not have a willing partner to give you a massage, never fear — you can do this yourself. Foot massage can be performed on dry feet, or you can oil your feet slightly using any vegetable oil and a drop or two of your favorite essential oil.

Step 1: Stroking stimulates circulation and warms the foot. Holding your partner's foot in your hands, on the top of the foot begin a long, slow, firm stroking motion with your thumbs, starting at the tips of the toes and sliding back away from you, all the way to the ankle; then retrace your steps back to the toes with a lighter stroke. Repeat this step three to five times. Now firmly stroke the bottom of the foot with your thumbs, starting at the base of the toes and moving from the ball of the foot over the arch, to the heel, and then back again. Repeat this step three to five times.

Step 2: Ankle rotations will loosen the joints and relax the feet. Cup one hand under the heel, behind the ankle, to brace the foot and leg. Grasp the ball of the foot with the other hand and turn the foot slowly at the ankle three to five times in each direction. With repeated foot massages, any stiffness will begin to recede. This is a particularly good exercise for those suffering from arthritis.

Step 3: Toe pulls and squeezes can be unbelievably calming, because toes are quite sensitive. Grasp the foot beneath the arch. With the other hand and beginning with the big toe, hold the toe with your thumb on top and index finger beneath. Starting at the base of the toe, slowly and firmly pull the toe, sliding your fingers to the top and back to the base. Now repeat, but gently squeeze and roll the toe between your thumb and index finger, working your way to the tip and back to the base. Repeat on the remaining toes.

Step 4: Toe slides are also very soothing. Grasp the foot behind the ankle, cupping under the heel. With the index finger of the other hand, insert your finger between the toes, sliding it back and forth three to five times.

Step 5: The arch press releases tension in the inner and outer longitudinal arches. Hold the foot as you did in step 4. Using the heel of your other hand, push hard as you slide along the arch from the ball of the foot toward the heel and back again. Repeat five times. This part of the foot can stand a little extra exertion, but don't apply too much pressure.

Step 6: Stroking is a good way to begin and end a foot massage. Repeat step 1.

The way to health is to have an aromatic bath and a scented massage every day.

— Hippocrates

Take a Luxurious Milk Bath

Why not use the skin-pampering benefits of milk by bathing in it instead of drinking it? Milk includes many components, such as proteins and fats, that are particularly good for soothing and moisturizing the skin.

• **To relieve itchy skin** due to sunburn or poison ivy or oak irritation, add 1 cup of instant, powdered whole milk and 1 cup of baking soda to running bathwater. Step in and soak for 15 minutes.

• **Make a milk-bath bag.** In a medium-size muslin drawstring bag or in a 12-inch square of doubled cheese-cloth, place 1 cup of instant, powdered whole milk, ½ cup of borax, ¼ cup of ground lavender flowers, and ¼ cup of ground rose petals. Tie the ends together or wrap with an elastic band. Drop into the tub as it fills with water, step in, and rub the bag over your skin to soften and lightly scent.

• **To combat dry, super-sensitive skin** or to bathe an infant's delicate skin, add 1 cup of instant, powdered whole milk; ¼ cup of finely ground raw almonds, pine nuts, walnuts, or pecans; and ¼ cup of marsh mallow root powder to a bath bag (see above). Drop into the tub as it fills with water, step in, and rub the bag over your skin.

Aromatherapeutic Milk Bath

Try this version of Cleopatra's famous bathing ritual and see whether your skin doesn't feel softer and smoother.

- 1 cup instant, powdered whole goat's or cow's milk
- 1 tablespoon apricot kernel, jojoba, avocado, hazelnut, or extra-virgin olive oil
- 8 drops essential oil of German or Roman chamomile, lavender, rosemary, spearmint, or rose

Pour the powdered milk and oil together directly under running bathwater. Add the essential oil immediately before you step into the tub. Swish with your hands to mix. Now relax!

Cleanse and Condition Your Complexion

Simple, natural cleansing creams, fruit pastes, and grain blends can be used to effectively and economically remove makeup and everyday dirt and grime that collects in your pores. Unlike soap — which has a tendency to dry the skin's surface — these products are very gentle and nourishing and do a thorough job of cleansing without stripping your skin of its natural barrier of protective oils.

Restore the Radiance

• **For smooth, soft skin,** wash your face every day with plain, organic yogurt or buttermilk. Use it as you would ordinary cold cream, avoiding the eye area. It's gentle enough for all skin types and as a bonus, it contains naturally occurring lactic acid. This acts as a mild exfoliant to remove dead-skin buildup.

• **For positively glowing skin,** mash a third of a very, very ripe banana in a small bowl. Use the pulp to wash your

All-Purpose Cleanser

This was my first-ever homemade cleansing formula. It naturally cleanses skin of excess oils, makeup, and dirt without drying, making it suitable for all skin types, even sensitive. (See page 14 for information on grinding ingredients.)

½ cup ground oatmeal
⅓ cup finely ground sun-
   flower seeds
¼ cup finely ground almond
   meal
Dash cinnamon (optional)

1 teaspoon powdered pep-
   permint or rosemary
   leaves, rose petals, or
   lavender flowers
Water, 1 or 2 percent milk,
   or heavy cream to moisten

1. In a medium-size bowl, mix all of the dry ingredients thoroughly.

2. Using approximately 2 teaspoons of scrub mixture for your face and throat, or more for your body, add enough water (for oily skin), milk (for normal skin), or heavy cream (for dry skin) to form a spreadable paste. Allow to thicken for 1 minute. Massage onto your face and throat or body area. Rinse.

3. Store any remaining blend in a zipper-lock plastic bag or plastic food container in the freezer for up to a year.

face and throat, avoiding the eye area. If your skin is especially dry or dehydrated, leave this on for approximately 5 minutes. Rinse, then pat dry.

• **To pamper mature, thin, dry skin,** mix 1 tablespoon of heavy cream with 1 or 2 drops of essential oil of rose or rose geranium. Use as you would a cleansing lotion, massaging well into your face and throat. This can be used on the eye area to remove eye makeup and mascara. This blend smells exquisite and if a drop happens to drip into your mouth, it will taste like a rose shake!

Keep Your Pearly Whites Gleaming

Most dentifrices today contain harsh abrasives, saccharin, sugar, detergents, and bleaches. Combine these ingredients with the twice-daily use and misuse of toothbrushes and the result is extra wear and tear on tooth enamel and gum tissue. You can make effective and pleasant natural dentifrices that will leave your teeth sparkling and your gums in the pink.

Herbal Toothpaste

A great alternative to commercial sweetened toothpastes! This recipe yields about 10 applications.

- 4 teaspoons baking soda
- 1 teaspoon finely ground sea salt
- 1 teaspoon myrrh powder
- 1 teaspoon white cosmetic clay
- 2 tablespoons vegetable glycerin
- 10 drops essential oil of orange, tea tree, rosemary, anise, lemon, spearmint, or peppermint

In a small bowl, thoroughly blend all ingredients until a spreadable paste forms. Store in a small jar. Dip a dry toothbrush into the mixture and brush normally.

Step Back, Plaque

• In a small bowl, combine 1 teaspoon of baking soda with 1 drop of essential oil of orange, lime, spearmint, or cinnamon. Dip a wet toothbrush into this mixture and brush your teeth as usual to fight plaque buildup and neutralize mouth odor.

• **Try strawberries for a brighter smile!** Mash a very ripe strawberry into a pulp. Dip your toothbrush into the pulpy liquid and brush normally. Strawberries have a slight bleaching action. Rinse thoroughly after brushing.

• **Out on a weekend camping trip** and forgot your toothbrush? Peel a 3- or 4-inch twig freshly cut from a sweet gum or flowering dogwood tree and chew on the end until it is frayed and soft. Now gently rub your teeth and gums. The twig can also be dipped in water and baking soda, if you desire.

Find Time for Fitness

What's the first thing to go when your daily schedule gets overburdened? For most people, it's physical exercise. But exercise helps you deal effectively with the physical and psychological demands of a hectic life. How do you find more time — or use the time you have more wisely — to get healthy, toned, and trim?

Exercise Is Essential

• **Break up your exercise routine** into 10-minute segments and try to fit three to six segments into your day. The benefits are practically the same as if you were to do just one long routine.

• **Find a better way to commute to work.** If possible, walk or ride your bicycle. If that isn't possible, park a mile or two away from work and hoof it to the office. If you take a train or bus, get off at the stop prior to your regular one. Your legs will soon reflect all this added mileage!

• **Find creative new ways to integrate family time** with exercise. If you have children, don't just be a bystander at the local park or playground; get up and climb the jungle gym with them, or run around the bases playing softball. Push a jogging stroller and give Junior a fun ride. Try bicycling, hiking, swimming, or just walking around the neighborhood with your family. Everyone will be healthier as a result.

- **Schedule your exercise time.** Make it a priority and stick to your commitment just as you would a scheduled doctor's or dentist's appointment.

- **Work out first thing in the morning.** I find that if I get my exercise finished and out of the way, I don't have to try to fit it in at the end of the day when I'm usually tired and might be tempted to skip my workout altogether.

- **Combine work with exercise.** Sound strange? I love to in-line skate, and while I'm whizzing up and down my neighborhood streets, I carry a small tape recorder and make notes. My neighbors thought I was a bit strange at first, but they're used to me now. You can do this as you walk, also.

Health is something we do for ourselves, not something that is done to us; a journey rather than a destination; a dynamic, holistic, and purposeful way of living.

— Dr. Elliott Dacher

• **Make dinner while you exercise.** If you enjoy one-pot dinners or main-course casseroles, pop one on the stove or into the oven and do your workout while it cooks. A Crock-Pot is a real blessing for busy people. It cooks slowly and for a long time so you can do other things while making dinner. As a bonus, exercising before you eat may take the edge off your appetite — and boost your metabolism, too.

• **Make exercise time your time.** There's no better way to pamper yourself than by taking care of your health.

Eat High-Energy Snacks

In the mood for a snack? Need fast food that will satisfy your cravings without empty calories and fat? Here are a few of my favorite delicious, guilt-free, quick snacks.

Need a Boost?

• **For a high-protein snack,** top melba toast or a rice cake with peanut or sesame butter or cottage cheese.

Sweet-and-Nutty Snack Mix

Convenient and portable, this mix is 100 percent better for you than a candy bar or chips! You'll get approximately 3½ cups from this recipe.

½ cup raw almonds
½ cup raw hazelnuts
½ cup dried, unsulfured, pitted cherries
½ cup large, unsulfured raisins
½ cup raw Brazil nuts
¼ cup lightly salted sunflower seeds, toasted
¼ cup lightly salted pumpkin seeds, toasted
¼ cup dried, unsulfured apricots, chopped
¼ cup carob or chocolate chips (optional)
Dash cinnamon or nutmeg (optional)

Place all ingredients in a plastic bag or food storage container and shake well. Keep tightly sealed in the refrigerator unless consumed within two weeks; raw nuts become rancid quicker than roasted ones. Consume a handful or so whenever the snacking mood strikes.

- **For a super-cooling summertime snack,** nothing beats sweet, frozen, seedless grapes. They're a tasty, crunchy treat that's full of vitamins and minerals.

- **Fight the midafternoon attack** of the Munch Monster by eating one of my favorite snacks — medjool dates. Slice a large date in half, remove the pit, insert a raw pecan into each half, then sprinkle with coconut flakes.

- **To organic plain yogurt or fortified soy yogurt,** add any or all of the following: ripe raspberries, blackberries, sliced peaches, strawberries, kiwi, papaya, almond slivers, raisins, and granola. Stir well and drizzle with honey or maple syrup, if desired.

Harness the Power of Your Shower

Turn your ordinary daily cleansing shower into a therapeutic spa. While a tub full of warm, sudsy, aromatic water conjures thoughts of relaxation, a shower can offer a wide array of body-pampering benefits simply by concentrating the flow of water onto specific body parts, enabling you to tackle problems such as sore muscles, headache, low energy, and lackluster hair, to name a few.

Hydrotherapies

• **Increase Your Energy:** Shower in water that's approximately body temperature for 2 to 3 minutes, then lower the temperature to very cool for about 15 to 30 seconds. Repeat this procedure twice more. Incidentally, this form of hydrotherapy has been used for centuries by many cultures to strengthen the immune system, thereby staving off colds and flus.

• **Hydrate Scaly Skin:** For skin that resembles a desert reptile's, take a quickie shower for about 2 minutes in warm water. While your skin is still wet, slather on your favorite body oil, then pat dry.

• **Head Off a Headache:** A handheld shower apparatus is best for this type of therapy. Turn on very warm water and aim the stream directly onto the aching area of your head for 5 minutes. Frequently, simply aiming the water onto the back of your head and neck will ease the pain. Some people find that alternating very warm and cold water every 30 seconds for 5 minutes works wonders, too.

• **Reduce Swelling:** To reduce inflammation to an acute injury such as a burn, sprained ankle or wrist, or severely stubbed toe, aim a cold spray of water onto the affected part for 5 minutes, then off for 5 minutes, repeating a few times. Do this immediately after the injury occurs, then seek medical attention if necessary.

• **Relieve Sore Muscles:** For muscles that are chronically sore or are sore from mere overexertion, but are not inflamed, aim a very warm water spray directly onto the muscle(s) for 5 minutes, then off for 5 minutes. Do this a few times.

• **Put an End to PMS Pain:** To relieve lower-back pain occurring before or during menstruation, I find that a very warm stream of water concentrated on my lower back for a few minutes helps lessen the cramping and muscle tension. Follow with a rich moisturizer to avoid dry skin.

Condition Your Tresses

Most men and women today style their hair to some degree daily. Whether it's simply a quick blow-dry or a complex ritual of moussing, drying, using hot rollers, brushing, then topping it all off with hair spray, your hair takes a lot of abuse.

Consider, too, environmental stress. Sunshine, salt water, chlorine, cigarette smoke, pollution, and dry office air all take their toll — hair is not meant to take this kind of constant torture.

Restore Your Crowning Glory

The following recipes are quite simple to make and, with consistent use, they will improve the condition of your hair and scalp.

Tressonaise

Smooth your mane with this recipe for homemade mayonnaise filled with hair-healthy conditioning ingredients that will add shine and softness.

    1 whole egg plus 1 egg yolk (room temperature)
 1½ tablespoons lemon juice
    1 cup unrefined olive, avocado, or sesame oil

1. Put the eggs and lemon juice in a blender and blend on medium, covered, for 5 seconds. Remove the cover and begin to drizzle the oil in a slow, steady stream. The mayonnaise should now be thick.

2. Store in a covered, glass container in the refrigerator. This recipe makes one treatment for long hair, two treatments for shoulder-length hair, or three treatments for short hair.

3. Apply enough mayonnaise to dry hair to cover the damaged parts. If you have an oily scalp but dry, frizzy, damaged ends, then treat only the lower portion of your hair. Cover your hair with a shower cap or plastic bag, then wrap with a warm towel. Leave on for up to an hour, then shampoo once or twice to remove all traces of oil. You may use once a week, if desired.

• **To condition dry, brittle, damaged hair,** mash a very ripe, large banana. Add a tablespoon each of heavy cream and honey and whisk together until smooth. Apply to dry hair from the roots to the ends, cover with a shower cap, and then wrap your head with a warm towel. Allow the mixture to remain on your hair for as long as possible — up to an hour. Rinse thoroughly with warm water, then shampoo as usual. If necessary, follow with a natural, detangling light conditioner.

• **Enhance the gloss of normal or dry hair** with jojoba oil. Actually a plant wax, not an oil, this yellow substance closely resembles human sebum. It makes a superb scalp and hair conditioner. To 6 tablespoons of jojoba oil, add 1 teaspoon each of the following essential oils: rosemary, basil, lemon, and lavender. Store in a 4-ounce, dark glass bottle. Shake vigorously before each use. Use within one year for maximum potency. Apply 1 or 2 tablespoons to dry hair and scalp. There's no need to soak your hair; just make sure all the strands are coated thoroughly. Be sure to give your scalp a good 5-minute massage to stimulate circulation and encourage hair growth. Cover your head with a shower cap and wrap with a warm, damp towel for up to an hour. Shampoo and follow with a good, light detangling conditioner if necessary. This treatment may be used weekly.

• **Rinse, rinse, rinse.** If smooth and silky hair is your aim, proper rinsing is crucial. Even the best conditioners will leave your hair drab and dull if they are not rinsed out completely.

Learn Anti-aging Secrets

The search for the ever-elusive Fountain of Youth is still going strong. This is evidenced by the scores of commercials advertising the sale of anti-wrinkle creams, skin-lightening creams, energy-boosting nutrition supplements, and memory-enhancing herbal products, not to mention the increasing popularity of plastic surgery.

The way I see it, true youthfulness can't be purchased in a bottle or from a doctor. But the attributes of youth — smooth skin, an alert mind, an active, limber body — can be prolonged into old age if you adhere to a youthful lifestyle and use common sense.

Maintain a Youthful Lifestyle

• **The old adage,** "Early to bed, early to rise, makes you healthy, wealthy, and wise," still rings true today. Getting plenty of high-quality, sound sleep allows your body to rest, recharge, repair, and replenish so you'll be rarin' to go the next day.

• **Stimulate your brain.** Don't allow yourself to become bored with life. Pick up a new hobby, find a new challenge, go back to school, read more. You *can* teach an old "dog" new tricks!

• **Become a "people person."** Reach out and try to help someone every day.

- **Slow down; pace yourself.** Quit scurrying around like a squirrel preparing its nest for winter. You can't enjoy life if you run through it at breakneck speed.

- **Get a pet.** Studies show that pet owners live healthier, happier, less stressful lives.

- **Hydrate your skin.** Dry skin ages prematurely, exhibiting lines and wrinkles long before Mother Nature intended. Apply a good moisturizing lotion morning and evening. Don't forget eight glasses of pure water daily, too!

- **Wear sunscreen.** Nothing ages your skin faster than the sun's rays. Sun damage is cumulative. That golden tan of youth will eventually produce unwelcome wrinkles, uneven pigmentation, age spots, and potentially skin cancer in your later years.

- **Eat fresh, whole, unprocessed foods.** Avoid empty-calorie, junky, chemical-laden foods. They do nothing but satisfy a temporary craving. Real food satisfies your soul and truly nourishes your body.

- **Exercise daily.** Use it or lose it! A sedentary lifestyle contributes to obesity, cardiovascular problems, stiff joints, lackluster skin and hair, and low energy — all signs of old age.

- **Keep a positive attitude.** Negativity affects not only your mood, your job performance, your physical appearance, and your health in general, but the people around you as well. No one wants to be around a person with low self-esteem.

- **Simplify your life.** It's not the material things in life that bring true happiness, it's friends, family, good food, pets, and time spent doing things you most enjoy.

Stay Cool and Dry

Natural body and foot powders are a chemical-free way to fight odor and perspiration. You can easily make your own customized body powders that will keep you cool and dry all day long.

Lavender Powder

This is a delightfully soft, silky body powder. The recipe makes about 1⅛ cups.

- ½ cup white cosmetic clay, arrowroot, or cornstarch
- ¼ cup powdered lavender flowers
- ¼ cup powdered rose petals
- 1 tablespoon zinc oxide powder
- ½ teaspoon essential oil of lavender
- 10 drops essential oil of rose (optional)

Mix the dry ingredients in a large bowl or food processor. Add the essential oils a few drops at a time and thoroughly incorporate into the powder. Store this in a special shaker container or recycled spice jar. Use within one year.

Herbal Body and Foot Powders

Some excellent base-powder choices to use alone or in combination include cornstarch, rice flour, arrowroot, French clay, white cosmetic clay, powdered calendula flowers, and powdered chamomile flowers. Customize your powder by adding your favorite essential oils or powdered flowers. Powders are simple to formulate and are great gifts.

• **My favorite mixture** is 1 part cornstarch, 1 part arrowroot, and 1 part powdered calendula flowers. This mixture makes for a very light powder — perfect for infants.

• **To keep your feet cool, dry, and odor-free,** try this blend: Combine ½ cup of baking soda, 2 tablespoons of zinc oxide powder, 2 tablespoons of white cosmetic clay, ½ cup of arrowroot, and 1 teaspoon of essential oil of orange, geranium, or peppermint. If you have athlete's foot or particularly odoriferous feet, substitute ½ teaspoon each of essential oil of tea tree and thyme. To make, follow the directions in the recipe on page 55. Sprinkle into your shoes and socks once or twice daily.

• **For those with allergies,** a powder made from 100 percent arrowroot powder, cornstarch, or white cosmetic clay will generally be irritation-free.

Cultivate Some Zzzzzzzzzzs

Has your get-up-and-go got up and gone? Suffering from brain fog? Too much on your mind to relax? Feeling constantly cranky? Insomnia a problem lately? Sleep deprivation takes its toll on both your face and your body in a hurry. To look and feel your absolute best, you need to get approximately seven to nine hours of deeply restful, quality sleep each night.

"Perchance to Dream . . ."

• **Flannel sheets are an insomniac's best friend!** Year-round, I sleep between thick, 6-ounce flannels that feel like light, soft, velvety blankets of fluffy cotton. During hot summer weather, forgo the usual thin blanket and substitute the top flannel sheet as your cover.

• **Get plenty of vigorous exercise early in the day** so you'll be naturally tired come bedtime. Exercise performed too close to retiring can be too stimulating for some people.

> *There must be stillness for the spirit to enter.*
>
> —Anonymous

• **Sip a cup of hot catnip, chamomile, or raspberry leaf herbal tea.** Hot, mineral-rich vegetable broth, cow's milk, and calcium-fortified soy or rice milk are also good. Drink it an hour prior to bedtime or you'll wake up needing to visit the lavatory.

• **Don't go to bed on a full stomach.** Digestion takes lots of energy and will keep you awake.

• **Go to bed at the same time every night.** Once your body gets used to a routine, it will naturally want to fall asleep at the designated time.

• **Put a drop or two of soothing essential oil** of lavender or Roman chamomile on your pillow.

• **Purchase a device** that drowns out disturbing noises and produces sleep-inducing sounds such as ocean waves lapping the shore, a gently babbling brook, or wind in the trees.

• **Avoid caffeinated products** such as certain brands of pain relievers, diet pills, and the usual culprits — coffee, cola drinks, chocolate, and black tea. Caffeine keeps you awake, makes for more restless sleep, and acts as a diuretic, causing you to make more trips to the bathroom.

Sleepytime Balm

So simple to make, yet so effective. Gentle enough to safely pacify even the most irritable, restless infant.

  ¼ cup all-vegetable shortening (room temperature)
  10 drops essential oil of orange
  2 drops essential oil of ylang-ylang
  1 drop essential oil of vanilla (optional)

Combine all ingredients in a small bowl and whip together using a small spatula or whisk. Apply a dab of balm to your temples after cleansing your face and just prior to bedtime. Use daily, if desired. Store in a 2-ounce plastic or glass jar in a dry, cool place for up to three or four months.

Make Your Own Bath and Massage Oils

Bath and massage oils are very easy to make at home. You simply need a base oil and any essential oil you desire. I like to use jojoba oil as my base because it does not need refrigeration and will not go rancid. Grapeseed, apricot kernel, and hazelnut oils also make great base oils because they are very light, but they must be refrigerated.

Soften and Scent Your Skin

• **Uplifting, Energizing Oil:** Combine 1 tablespoon of jojoba oil with 2 drops each of essential oils of peppermint, rosemary, and eucalyptus. Add to your bath while the tap is running. For a deodorizing foot treatment, have a friend massage your clean, tired feet with the oil for 15 minutes. Then put on socks, and go to bed.

• **Exotic Oil:** This formula conditions dry skin and leaves a sensual, musky fragrance. Mix 1 cup jojoba oil with ¼ teaspoon each of these essential oils: sandalwood, patchouli,

Nourishing Oil

This vitamin- and mineral-rich formula is good for all skin types, especially normal and dry. Excellent for dry, ragged cuticles, too.

- 1 tablespoon *each* of the following oils:
  almond, apricot kernel, avocado, hazelnut, jojoba, and extra-virgin olive oil
- 1,200 international units (IUs) vitamin E oil (d-alpha tocopherol)

Combine all ingredients in an 8-ounce glass or plastic bottle. Tightly cap and shake vigorously. Store in the refrigerator for up to a year. For your bath, add 2 teaspoons to running water. For massage, use directly on your skin as needed.

and vetiver. Then add ¼ teaspoon of synthetic musk oil (optional). Store away from heat and light in a tightly sealed, 8-ounce, dark glass bottle. To use, add 2 teaspoons to the bath while the tub is filling. For massage, use ½ teaspoon of essential oil blend to ½ cup of jojoba oil.

Pamper Those Peepers

It's said that the eyes are the windows to the soul. But if you look at a computer screen all day, party all night, spend time around smokers or in dry office air, have allergies, or forget to remove your mascara, your "windows" are going to look puffy, bloodshot, or irritated, or they'll have dark circles beneath them. They may even sting and tear.

Add Sparkle to Your Eyes

Your eyes are your most expressive features — do your best to pamper them. Follow these suggestions to soothe, brighten, and refresh red and weary eyes.

• **Pep up your pretty peepers** with plenty of sound sleep — one of the best beautifiers there is!

• **Swollen eyes and dark circles** can sometimes be the result of toxin buildup in the body, as well as dehydration. When the body is dehydrated, the kidneys try to retain water, which results in puffiness. Drink plenty of water daily in order to flush toxins and excess sodium from your body. The more water you drink, the less you will retain.

• **For swollen eyelids,** dip cotton balls or cosmetic squares into icy-cold whole milk or cream. Lie down, and apply soaked cotton to your eyelids. Leave on for 5 to 10 minutes. The high fat content of either liquid provides a moisturizing treatment for the delicate, thin skin around your eyes.

• **Tune out. Don't be a TV addict.** The glare from the screen is not good for your eyes. Besides, you can spend your time more wisely.

• **See your way clear** by eliminating sore, dry, red, irritated eyes. My favorite treatment is to keep handy a bottle of lavender aromatic hydrosol and spritz my face and eyes with it as often as necessary. The liquid is so pure and gentle that I can spray it directly into my opened eyes. I find it extremely soothing. German chamomile and rose hydrosol work equally well.

• **Apply a chilled, water-based lotion** or gel around the eye area once a day after cleansing to moisturize the delicate skin. A cucumber-based product is a good choice.

• **A daily application of sunscreen** to the skin around your eyes is essential if you want to prevent sun damage and the formation of dark circles. Choose a product specifically designed to be used on the face.

• **Add 2 or 3 drops of essential oil** of calendula to a small jar of chilled herbal eye cream. The resulting bright orange cream will help offset the blue color of dark circles, and the calendula essential oil is guaranteed to restore and soothe tired eyes, leaving them revived and refreshed.

• **Out of eye makeup remover?** Apply a dab of all-vegetable shortening to the eye area and gently rub over your lashes. It will dissolve even the most stubborn water-proof mascara and eyeliner. Makes a great impromptu moisturizer for dry patches of eczema and psoriasis, too!